BODY MIND TRANSFORMATIONS
Lessons and Insights to Create
The Best Version of YOU

FORREST FOLEN, SHELTON MATSEY, MATT JENNINGS, SAMANTHA NICOLE, SAMAN BAKHTIAR, RACHEL RICHARDS, MOLLY KUBES, BOB THOMPSON, ANTHONY STEEL

FOREWORD
LISA NICHOLS

Table of Contents

FOREWORD
LISA NICHOLS

First of all, let me be clear that I'm writing this forward NOT as a physical fitness trainer or specialist, but as a woman who has been on a tumultuous fitness journey for years. While one year I felt like the victor over my fitness and the next year, I would feel like the victim. Navigating through my own fitness journey over the past 25 years has allowed me to witness the industry from multiple viewpoints.

We've seen a well-intentioned fitness community for years express the importance of eating healthy, staying fit, and keeping active. And for years, we've been given the tools - the exercises, the gym memberships, the kettlebells, the yoga mats, the green shakes, the special diets, the workout DVD's, and even the "Brazilian booty " programs - but why on earth hasn't anything changed?
Many of us have even gone as far as to do whatever it takes to lose weight, even when it directly compromises our health -, pills, fasting, binge-cardio, saunas with sweaters on. Let's be real, I've tried many of these myself.

…And let's also be real and say that sometimes medical intervention is absolutely necessary when it could be a life or death situation, so there's absolutely no shame in that.

But we all know we don't have to hit a rock bottom to start climbing a mountain, so let's commit together in making a change RIGHT NOW.

REMEMBER - You can do this!

I battled with being over 210 pounds for 17 years. On the outside my life was soaring with bestselling book after book, international speaking gigs and a company that grew astronomically year after year. However, my everyday success high and excitement was matched with an everyday sadness and shame. If I looked to some as a superwoman then I felt as if my battle with my weight was my kryptonite.

My goal isn't to hype anything up. My goal is to help you realize that just because something didn't work for you in the past, doesn't mean it's worth giving up.

Would you give up on your kids? Would you give up on your parents? What about on your friends?

Of course not!

So why would you even consider giving up on yourself?

We all know WHAT to do, but it's worth investigating - why don't we actually take the time to do what we already know?

We all know that food like brown rice, avocado, and broccoli are good for us! Walking more, drinking more water, and exercise are all things we should be doing regularly. I've questioned for a long time now if a new gym membership or a new "quick-fix diet" is really the answer we need, when what we're after is: A permanent, well-balanced solution to staying lean, fit, and healthy.

Going through my own wellness journey, I'm all too familiar with the emotional roller coaster. I can tell you, it's absolute madness what we put ourselves through. I'm all too familiar with the shame, the hurt, and the guilt. To top it off, we keep piling on the shame, failure after failure, and then we cover it up in what we eat with the "comfort foods" that help make us feel better in the moment. How ironic is that!?

The truth is, there's no "one-size-fits-all, cookie cutter" approach that's going to work for every BODY. We all need to search for the key to our own health and fitness lifestyle. The best program for you is the one you can stick to, and it's the

MINDSET, not the program, that will get you to where you want to go in the end.

…and that's exactly what the experts and authors in this BODY MIND TRANSFORMATIONS BOOK set out to do for you - establish the MINDSET for long-term success.

Unless we deal with the root cause of WHY we became out of shape, overweight, and unfit, and WHY we must succeed NO MATTER WHAT, we'll never truly create a solution for ourselves that will last.

For me, I finally evolved to understand that after being a state champion athlete in high school and thirteen years of sports that my unwanted weight was an 80 pound jacket for me. Something that covered my true essence and kept me safe from all of the physical attention that I was unable to manage in my twenties. And it also "helped" me to make more immediate connections with women with more ease and without what previously felt like harsh judgment. I did achieve my goal in minimizing the attention to me and eliminating a barrier between me and connecting with other women. But I also traded in a short term social challenge with a long-term personal nightmare. I thought that It was all a physical thing, "Lisa just one more diet, Lisa just get more aggressive stronger pills." I never considered that it was a mind AND body journey, after all, I was already Motivating the Masses right? Wrong! Even though I was traveling the globe inspiring millions to live their best live, I needed to become my own rescue.

Each of the transformational coaches in this book has a slightly different approach, but they all stick with the common theme which is that your success will happen when you apply your BODY and the MIND together into making a TRANSFORMATION.

I encourage you to move through this book wearing a new outfit, and I'm not talking about gym clothes here. I strongly encourage you to wear an outfit like Indiana Jones… the outfit of an adventurer, who seeks new and exciting ways of looking at fitness, and at yourself.

Like I wrote about in detail in my book, "Abundance NOW", I spent 17 years of my life not wholeheartedly loving the skin I was in. However, when I made my health non-negotiable and acquired the right mindset to success, I was finally able to take off the 80-pound jacket I was in. If I was able to make my fitness journey a success, I know that with the tools and the inspiration you'll find in this book that you can, too.

The holistic approach of bringing in to play your complete self - body, mind, and spirit is what this book is all about, and if you're ready, or better yet, even if you're not ready but you are willing, then let's go on this journey and commit to our greatest health together.

Last, before you jump in, I encourage you wholeheartedly to leave the guilt and shame behind. If you're like I once was, you've probably excelled at putting everyone else first, and putting yourself last. However, once you put yourself first, you'll see that now you have the strength to help everyone else without burning out or building resentment.

We cannot change our last chapter, as it has already been written in ink. But we can change the way our next chapter will be written because we are still holding the pen in our hands.

Yours Sister in Abundance, Health, and Prosperity,

~Lisa Nichols
www.motivatingthemasses.com

THE PATH TO YOUR BEST LIFE
FORREST FOLEN

I've been a fitness pro and mindset and meditation coach for over 17 years. I've founded 2 successful fitness companies, I've helped thousands of people transform their health and their lives with a holistic body, mind, and spirit approach, I'm a 2nd degree Black Belt in Tae Kwon Do, I've trained for over 10 years with a meditation master, I've been featured on Oprah Winfrey and Deepak Chopra's newsletter, and I'm also an international best-selling author.

However, I wasn't always the body, mind, and spirit and mindset coach people know me as today.

When I was in my teens I fell onto a path of smoking, doing drugs, drinking, and self-destructive behaviors.

*I go into full detail in my book, "Awakening To Your Fitness Journey" by Forrest Folen and Anthony Steel.

It got so bad that for a time, I ended up homeless and hopeless.

Luckily for me, when I hit that rock-bottom moment, I was given some sage advice by my grandmother.

She told me, *"Forrest, take care of your body. If you take care of your body, your body will take care of your mind, and your mind will take care of your life"*.

This simple "grandmother blueprint" literally saved my life and became the guiding principle on how I lived my life from then on and why I shared my passion of fitness and mindset with so many others over the course of the last 2 decades.

Of course I've made many mistakes along the way, but a major lesson I've taken away from one of my mentors is to continue failing forward. Mistakes are part of the path to success. In fact, when someone told Thomas Edison he failed 1,000 times when trying to invent the lightbulb he told them that on the contrary he didn't fail, he actually discovered 1,000 ways not to create a light bulb!

Perspective is everything.

Your perspective holds in it your version of the truth. Not THE truth, but YOUR truth. And in your truth you have your accumulation of life experiences, your perception of those experiences, beliefs about you and your life, and because of all those things have developed an expectation of what is possible in your life.

Now, living according to expectation isn't in itself a bad thing. However, for most people it ends up being the limiting factor of their life in one or more of the key spheres that matter.

The spheres of your life that matter are some of the following:

- Health
- Wealth
- Career
- Family life
- Romantic relationship
- Social life
- Spiritual life

There are others areas of life that matter as well, such as your education, your sex life, your hobbies, artistic expression, but we'll at least start here with the above list.

You may not have found a rock bottom in life such as I did, or you might feel like you're drowning and you've been tied to a rock and thrown into a river…either way you want to improve and you want to grow in life, correct?

Like most people, you want deeper connection in your relationships, you want to be fit and in optimal health, you want to live in a way that feels fulfilling to you, and you want the best for you and your family.

However, that can't happen without you getting past the one thing that will block and stop you in your tracks each and every time.

Do you know what the one thing that can stop you is?

Have you identified the limiting factor in your life from living to your potential?

Do you know what's keeping you from an abundance of happiness, fulfillment, money, love, and peace in your life?

The answer is…*YOU!*

You are the one who has the power to peel back the layers of your ego and live according to the person you truly are and to create the ideal version of yourself that you want to become.

The ego I'm referring to here is not your pride, and I'm not using the term ego as in the way of "you're an egotistical person". It's something different than that. The ego I'm referring to is your self image. Your ego is the view of who you think you are, constructed of years of life experience, viewpoints, and inferences, beliefs, traumas, and perspectives.

Your ego is not who you really are. It's who you *think* you really are.

Your ego is built of your conditioned self.

Your ego has been constructed by everything that has ever influenced you such as your culture, your parents, friends, religion, TV and news media, pop culture, life trauma, things people have said about you and the labels others or yourself have given you (You're fat, skinny, smart, pretty, ugly, determined, broke, rich, spoiled, inconsistent, hard-working, a bad person, angry, a loser, a champion, etc.).

There are some great things that can happen as a result of your ego, for instance labeling yourself a "hard worker" can create an image in you that drives you toward success.

However, the most important thing to know about ego is this. Ego is always more damaging than constructive, because it always comes with detriment to the Self and many times to other people involved in the path of the person who's ego has taken over in the drivers seat.

Ego-driven mentalities are ultimately the basis for all violence, war, killing, withholding of resources, abuse, exploitation, stealing, greed-based living, fear, suffering, and torment of the world.

By dissolving the layers of ego and living beyond the ego-driven life, we encompass the vast possibility of all that is good and true in life. We become connected with ourselves and others and live in accordance with our most natural state of being; a state of freedom in mind and in life.

The ego is never satisfied. It needs to feed. And it attaches to things that aren't the source of joy, but are the illusions of happiness and joy.

"You can't satisfy the ego. You can only feed it's hunger with ego snacks like thrills, chemicals, conceit, anger, gossip, purchases, and achievements. But, shortly after these feedings, the ego returns…larger and hungrier than before".

- Dean Jackson

The Ego = False Self

Me, me, me!, Separation, Blame, Hostility, Resentment, Pride, Complain, Jealousy, Anger, Power, Materialism, Madness, War, Coldness, Past/Future oriented, Intolerance, Self-importance, Egoism, Self-denial, Social intolerance, Living up to this and that, Doing, If I achieve "X", then I'll be happy.

The Non-Ego Self = True Self

We, Unity, Understanding, Friendliness, Forgiveness, Love, Gratefulness, Co-happiness, Happiness, Humble, Spiritualism, Wisdom, Peace, Sympathy and Empathy, Present moment oriented Tolerance, We-importance, Altruism, Self-acceptance, Social acceptance, Simplicity, Just be, Needs nothing to feel complete.

"Ego means self-identification with thinking, to be trapped in thought, which means to have a mental image of "me" based on thought and emotions. So ego is there in the absence of a witnessing presence."
- Eckhart Tolle

So the reason you're feeling like your weight or your health is a big problem that you can't overcome, or that you're having trouble with your spouse, or that your kids are driving you crazy, or that you're always so "busy" all the time, or that it seems you can never catch a break financially, or that you don't feel spiritually connected - any of this and more, is not because you need to *get something* in order to fulfill what you need.

The reason is that your EGO and the layers of beliefs you hold have stopped you from tapping into the possibilities that already exist within you and around you to achieve and become what and who you truly want.

In other words, you become trapped in the past. If all you've always gotten was a certain result, you'll continue to expect that result.

And if your future vision isn't exactly what you truly want, or if there's something in your vision that makes you put the brakes on every time you start seeing forward momentum, then it's your ego, your self-image, that's sabotaging you.

Do you have one foot on the gas pedal and the other foot on the brake?

Do you start to see success and then sabotage yourself?

Do you become trapped in overthinking and fear?

If you do, you're not alone. In fact, this IS the body, mind, spirit journey! The obstacles you face are exactly what you need right now in your life to become the strong person you are meant to become!

So the final question is HOW?

It's one thing to know WHAT the problem is, and as I've outlined, it's the limiting beliefs and mindset patterns of your ego; your conditioned self.

What we need to tap into is the non-ego self, your TRUE SELF. The good news is there is a process for this, and it's a proven process. This is the process I teach to my mindset coaching clients from all over the World.

When you tap into this version of you, you will create your best life. You'll see more opportunity and you'll become the type of person who will attract the people, circumstances, and events that will take you to where you want to go in life.

It takes a degree of guidance, coaching, and accountability to get there, but the basic steps I've outlined below.

7 Steps to Living a Non-Ego Driven, True Self Life - Your BEST Life!*

Step 1) Find your WHY - What's your motivation? What has been frustrating you or causing you pain? What does success look like to you? Once you can become clear on your "why" then you'll be motivated to stick with the process even when the going gets tough!

Step 2) Awareness - You first need to become aware of your thoughts, emotional patterns, habits, beliefs, to have the ability to make a change. The tricky thing is that almost everyone thinks they are 100% aware, UNTIL they start to study their own awareness!

Step 3) Acceptance - By accepting that what you experience is ONE PERSPECTIVE and a STORY of what is happening in your life, you break free of the ego-attachment to being trapped in your own thought-centered version of yourself - the ego.

Step 4) Accountability - This is the moment of choice, and with your awareness and acceptance you're now in a position of making a true choice instead of just remaining stuck in your past conditioning. By continually choosing the path that leads you to the best outcomes, you break free of ego-driven reactionary way of being to living in a state of present-moment consciousness, which leads to…

Step 5) Adaptation - A passive adaptation will occur as you practice this new method of present moment awareness. This is the adaptation that is a natural result of your being in a state of the observer, where you have the power to dissolve the false ego self and enter your highest self, the present-moment-oriented Self that is free from bound thoughts, feelings, and behaviors.

Step 6) Meditation - Practice entering the present moment. Break from the limiting ego mind and

16

move into a space of "no mind". From a practice of non-religious meditation your mind becomes clear, you release from the negative effects of stress, your emotions become balanced, and you break free from the ego that is controlling you and is the part of you that keeps you suffering and in bondage.

Step 7) Daily rituals - To succeed you must make your mindset training a daily practice. Just like exercise and nutrition, your results depend on your day-by-day habits and actions. Mindset training is no different. No matter how much you know or how much you think you know, it means nothing without consistency and perseverance. Establishing simple daily rituals is the final key to your long-term success.

*4 of the 7 steps above, the "4 A's" process, was taught to me by 2 of my mindset mentors, Brian Grasso and Carrie Campbell.

Our method of training comes from my experience training with over a dozen mindset coaches, mediation masters, and mentors. It's been proven hundreds upon hundreds of times to work each and every time as long as YOU have the right attitude.

In fact, the thing that changed my life the most was that I began seeing myself worthy as someone to invest time, energy, knowledge, mentorship and coaching in. I would have never achieved the level of success I have in my life today without my coaches - and that's why I recommend you find a coach. It doesn't have to be me, but you do need a coach, and it does have to be someone you resonate with.

Today I'm a father of 3 amazing kids. I've found the woman of my dreams who loves and supports me and who allows me to be myself. I'm healthy and happy. I have wonderful friends, family, and co-workers with whom I share my life. I live in a beautiful home by the beach in Southern California, and most of all I'm grateful to all the little things in life and I'm happy and fulfilled.

I want the same for you.

With a defeatist attitude you can't go very far. You have to be willing and able to extend trust, or at least try your best.

However, anyone with an attitude that displays a willingness to at least try…then the future is a bright one. Continue to take the path developing yourself as a person, and don't forget to love yourself exactly for who you are right now.

"Personal development is the belief that you are worth the effort, time, and energy needed to develop yourself". - Denis Waitley

~Forrest Folen
Find me on Facebook:
Forrest Folen
forrest@wayoflifetransformations.com.
www.wayoflifetransformations.com

TAILORED TO YOU
SHELTON MATSEY

What I have discovered working in the fitness industry is that every single person that I work with is an individual. There is no one-size-fits-all option when you are dealing with different people. There are some general concepts that, of course, work across the industry. However, until we look at our people as individuals and let them know how much we care; it becomes very difficult to get the results that our client wants and in the end. As a fitness professional, I want you to know that what we care about is you reaching the goal that you have in mind. My goal is to help you focus and create a goal that really is going to serve you.

I feel so blessed to be here today. I have been married for sixteen years. My wife Lyn and I have two amazing children. I am a fitness facility owner; of four locations. I have a kinesiology degree, which lead me into my personal training at Bally's Gym, as well as in school. I have a great team of coaches that help me work with over a thousand clients. Every day our focus, is not about getting more clients, it's about making sure that the ones that we have are getting the results that will really serve them.

I spent some time working the fitness industry, as a young man I worked at a Bally's fitness, and then I joined the Army and became an Air Defense Officer. I was Active Duty in the military for six years. During that time, got my MBA, and when I came out, I did what everyone expected me to do. I went to work for a large corporation. I made good money. I had the kind of job that everybody wants, but honestly, I did not like it. I often found myself drinking several bottles of mountain dew, eating sunflower seeds or even candy, to try to help myself to stay awake as I'm driving on the road getting to and from work. There was just no purpose in what I was doing, for me. When I combined that with the long days and the long commutes, I was not living a life that served me.

I remember in February of 2007, I ran into my old manager when I worked at Bally's, at the Chicago auto show. We talked, I told him what I had been up to, and he said "you should come over and check out what I'm doing." I said back to him at that point, I'm good, I'm where I'm supposed to be. We had recently bought a house, my wife was pregnant, and I was living what was supposed to be 'the right life.'

As the time went by, a couple of months later, I began to entertain the idea that maybe it really would be best if I moved on. What if what I'm doing, is not right for me? I know it's not what I want to do. My wife and I talked about it. We started by discussing what would happen if I did go back into the fitness industry? I would have to leave my steady job, my dependable income, and begin working in commissions, when I was not great at sales. In fact, I sucked at it. It was definitely not the safest or smartest answer, but something in me told me to do it. I knew it was a thing that I needed to do.

Even though my family told me that making that move was stupid, I took the leap in July. Calling my former Bally's manager and having him set me up an interview for where he was now working. I felt really nervous. I was, let's say, a little less than in the perfect condition I thought I should be in in order to do this new job efficiently. Physically, I wasn't horrible, but I didn't feel like I was really "in shape." It had been a while since I had done any training. I had a lot of fear as I walked into that interview, but I did get the job. Immediately, I began pouring myself into clients, my clients, learning all that I could do to make myself better for them.

 As a person; I'm reserved, I'm not really comfortable getting out there on the floor and selling, in fact, as I said before, I sucked at it, but I worked on it, I learned, and I had a good manager that gave me opportunities to grow and learn. I worked my way through because of all the new home stress due to not having that steady income anymore. I had bills that were going further and further into the rears, all the things that I was getting behind on, as I made this career, but I was happy now. I was enjoying what I was doing, and I was getting pretty good at it too, but the stress of everything at home, on top of the fear of failure that I felt every day. I continued to build my abilities and I eventually became one of the top trainers at that facility.

As I worked for them, I kept thinking to myself that I wanted to do more than just be out on the floor and getting more clients. How could I improve my surroundings? Why is it all about how many clients we have instead of how to help each client individually? How could I make things better for the clients? How could we help "Sally" lose that last 10 pounds or whatever it was to help her reach every one of her goals? Eventually I got tired of thinking about the hows and what ifs and I found a way to begin to start focusing on actually doing something about it all.

A friend of mine, one of my co-workers, and I started to collaborate in June of 2009. We scraped together a little bit of money, and started our own business. With our main vision of delivering results for the clients that we have, rather than focusing on just trying to get more clients. In general, in the fitness industry, they actually plan on not having everybody that they sign up, to actually show up. In fact, most of the facilities, if every single person showed up every day, they wouldn't be able to accommodate everyone.

I wanted to have a model that was based on helping people get the results, to show you that we care about who you are. I believe that attitude has shown up in everything that we do. We know our clients. We know their names, we know what is going on in their lives and by knowing this, it helps us to be able to help them have better results overall. A perfect example of that might be; if a client says that they want to reach this aggressive goal, but then we know that they have children who are in several sports or they have after school. They have so many different things that are going to be distractions to reaching this aggressive goal. So, we can then talk about the things that are in their life and ask whether this is the best goal for them, for where they are in their life. We find that our clients appreciate. They even have said to us, that they feel like family when they come into our location.

My wish is to really help people find what works for them. For one person, it may be a nutrition based plan that is just focused on clean eating and moderate carbs. For others, it might be lower carbs and higher protein. For some people, cardio really works for them because they love it, and others it's more about strength training. The key is finding whatever works for you. So that you can both live the lifestyle that you want to live, but also reach the fitness and nutrition goals that you both want and need in your life.

My goal to see in the fitness industry, not just my locations, is to move from the one-size-fits-all approach; in fitness and in nutrition. If we can work together to do that, as a team, we can find success. I have a goal to help transition the fitness industry, from something that is purely looking at you as someone to sell to, and begin to look at you as someone ready to take their life and their fitness seriously and make a difference one person at a time as we work with you to live your fit life.

~Shelton Matsey
Find me on Facebook:
Shelton Matsey
www.fitcodebootcamp.com

BACK TO BASICS: BUILDING STRENGTH
MATT JENNINGS

Being strong…It's important! It truly is. And with this short chapter I just want to share with you this theme: When we go the gym we are going there to get strong, not to lose weight.

Getting stronger will often have the side-effect of losing weight. But to focus on weight loss rather than the building of strength (and a little muscle) is a misbelief that we need to transition out of. The focus needs to be on building a foundation of strength and integrity in your body, and this cannot happen just doing cardio.

In the late 80's, and really throughout the 90's, the cardio and aerobics scene was blowing up. Why the fitness industry took such great interest in cardio and aerobics at this time, I'm not quite sure, but I would speculate that group fitness was certainly gaining some popularity. A typical group fitness class then may have been designed around a 3" step box, along with some dance moves choreographed to pop dance music, and a miked-up, leotard-clad instructor…and now we've got something. I'm not quite sure if that *something* was too effective, though. Maybe fun…yes. My wife Kathy was one of those prototypical aerobics class instructors of the late 80's and early 90's. She has mentioned that instructing and taking aerobics classes was indeed fun, yet looking back today, she agrees…not very effective after all. But I digress. The problem we nurtured for so long was that so many of us pushed cardio and aerobics as the top-dog means to an end, and did little in the way of investing some time building and sculpting our bodies where the iron lay.

Today, trainers and coaches are much more knowledgeable about how the body responds to the various ideals and methods concerning exercise. I will attest to one simple truth enveloping the beliefs of some of today's smartest and upcoming superstars in the gym biz world: strength training is the pervading principle behind every meaningful training routine/program in the western hemisphere of fitness. Why? Because it can make all of your dreams that drive you to go to the gym in the first place…come true.

Now, let's imagine for a moment that strength is a bucket. This bucket is where all the other cool things that are important in fitness are stored. Things like your aerobic capacity, anaerobic capacity, work capacity, strength endurance, power endurance, mobility, flexibility, athleticism, joint integrity…they can all be stored in that bucket of strength. Without strength as a bucket, there is limited storage to contain these other important qualities of fitness. Many of which can only be improved in the weight room.

In the fitness industry now, we have seen a turn towards a new narrative, where people who want to understand more of how to get the results they want from the time and effort they invest at the gym are spending more time at the squat rack (hopefully squatting), picking up somewhat heavy things off the ground, and putting somewhat heavy things overhead. It's so good to see programs and people in the gym environment moving towards this effective and essential approach. And as a coach of over 25 years, I have watched remarkable things come of it. Here is an example of what I mean by a scenario where "fitness dreams come true." Jenn has been a client of ours for about two years now. She has completed a couple of our 6 week body transformation challenges and assumed some fairly good results. She lost 36 pounds in twelve weeks which is outstanding. But during the next 8-9 months Jenn was a bit ebb and flow with her diet, and that is the probable reason she did not see even better results from her training during that post-challenge spread. But then again, Jenn was at the time interested in the scale and what it had to say about how things were going. Then one fateful Saturday Jenn came to one of our Strong-man/Strong-woman training sessions at the gym, where we typically pickup heavy things and move them or put them somewhere.

One of the exercises on this particular day was the Farmer Carry, where we load either two bars with some weighted plates, or what is called a "hex bar," which we load the same way. In this particular case, there were four hex bars from which to choose: one weighing 95 pounds…another 135 pounds…the third 185 pounds…and a fourth bar that weighed 225 pounds. Jenn picked up the 135 pound bar and immediately put it down. She then walked over to the 185 pound bar, picked it up, and walked with it for some twenty-or-so feet. She again put this bar down and looked at me somewhat curious and intrigued. Hmm…Jenn's not going to pick up the 225 pound beast I thought…is she?? Jenn then walked up to the bar weighing 225 pounds, set her feet, set her spine and braced before picking it up. She took in a big breath and pulled the bar off the ground and immediately walked one hundred feet before putting the bar back down. That simple (not easy) act of lifting something heavy and walking with it was a life changing moment for Jenn. I, as well as several others, watched and cheered her effort. A few hugs and more cheers celebrated Jenn truly taking her life to a whole new level.

Over the next several months, Jenn changed her focus on the type of training she did and the foods she put in her body. Instead of dieting to the muse of the scale, she focused on fueling her body to be strong and build muscle, all the while losing another forty pounds in the process.

Today, Jenn is a forty year old mom who has multiple Spartan Races, powerlifting events, and fitness shows under her belt. It's amazing how lifting a little weight can change the course of someone's life.

Here's one more quick story that is more about practicality than anything else. Years ago I trained a husband and wife team, let's call them Rick and Laura (why not…those are their real names). Laura would always get upset with me if we didn't do some type of 'cardio' exercise after our training sessions. Rick was good no matter what we did as he understood the training philosophy I believed in. On one particular day Laura got a little snippy with me and wanted to know exactly why I seemed so adverse to having them run more laps around the gym building, or having them do anything that got them all sweaty and collapsing a lung or two. Just for the record, I am not adverse to aerobic work, cardio, jogging or running from the invisible man just nipping at your heels. But this was my wise ass quip to her query: 'Let's say Laura that you, Rick and myself decided to go on a day hike on what begins as a beautiful, sunny and seemingly uneventful June day. We get several miles into our hike…let's make it ten miles, and suddenly a bolt of lightning strikes this big oak tree dropping a huge branch landing on me, pinning and shattering my leg (and me) to the ground. We are ten miles from any help…who is

going to help me?' Laura then says with a smirk…
'Well since I can run farther than Rick…I will get
you help' "Really?" I said… "By the time you run
away and find someone…and then find me …I have
likely bled to death. What I needed was for you to be
strong enough to help Rick get the giant tree branch
off of my leg." The long and short of this story would
be this: Most anyone can travel ten miles on foot on
most any given day. Yet how many are likely capable
of performing an act of strength enough to save
another's life?

Here is an idea I would like you to
consider…#LiftingIsCardio

~Matt Jennings
If there is anything I can help you with in your quest
for a stronger, sexier and better performing you,
please hit me up at matt@theliftgym.com
www.theliftgym.com

KEEPING YOUR VIBRATIONS HIGH TO BE AN ATTRACTIVE LEADER

SAMANTHA NICOLE

What does it mean to be an attractive leader? A leader who is passionate, magnetic and vibrant - the type that everyone seems to be drawn to follow because of their ability to stand within themselves with strength and knowing in their mission and message.

How do you become that leader? You have a mission and a message. You feel passionate and convicted by your purpose, but you're missing that element of magnetism. That energy that effortlessly draws people to work with you and for you. You've been experiencing burnout, exhaustion and that horrible sense that if you keep going at this pace, you're going to lose your heartfelt momentum.

Tony Robbins, a highly achieved entrepreneurial multi-billionaire, says that although there is a science to success, there is an art to fulfillment. When defining the art, we realize that there is no set-in-stone formula to deciding how one can feel fulfilled. It's different for every person and even for an individual, the requirements to feel good can change daily. All too often people take the proven steps to success and arrive to their destination feeling unhappy because they did not take the time to do the inner work of deciding what makes them feel good.

As a fitness coach for entrepreneurs, I have found that fulfilled success comes fastest when our energy is high. According to The Law of Attraction, you can attract anything you want by raising your energetic vibrations through feeling good. When you learn how to feel good, you open a pathway that allows you to constantly access your highest energy. Once a leader has accessed their highest energy, they truly become magnetic. They develop mental flexibility and emotional stamina. They become connected to their inner self and learn not to be thrown off by life's curveballs. This inner strength translates into true attractiveness and is what's sought after by people looking to learn from you.

Energetically, true magnetism, as defined by The Law of Attraction, is a byproduct of having high, aligned energy. When we are high energy individuals, when our vibrations are elevated, we become captivating. Since I train the physical body, I've learned that exercise is just a tool to access the strength of your inner being. Understanding how to fulfill your inner self develops the sense of confidence everyone is attracted to and has no relationship to the physical attraction that most focus on in order to be successful. Rather than the connotation of attraction that describes how you look externally, I want to redefine being attractive as being someone who has high vibrations coming from within. Just that by itself can magnetize people into your atmosphere because quite simply, they want to be around you. If you have good energy, you will attract anything that you desire in business; the right clients, increased income, brilliant ideas, and unstoppable motivation. Truly the options are limitless.

So why exercise? The way you assess your energetic attraction is by how in-tune you are with your body. Your body is ultimately - You. It holds awareness of where you stand with your emotions, your mentality and your capabilities. As you build a relationship with your body, you can learn to use fitness as a tool to train yourself into become more attractive. My wish for you is that you understand the value behind fitness, health and self-care, so that you can feel truly filled up as your reach your business goals daily.

Physically, through the process of working out, every hour you spend exercising, your endorphins rise and you become more self-aware. Kinesthetic awareness comes from spending time focusing on your body's movement, chemistry and response to outside influences. Because exercises can be challenging, relaxing, or taxing; the demands of these different energetic states is a training ground to teach your body how to respond, not react, to a variety of stressors. Whether you run, weight lift, or stretch; each scenario can offer you the opportunity to learn how to respond productively to your environment rather than react out of fear. Developing this energetic strength and flexibility is a large component of being a good leader. A more simple yet powerful physiological benefit, is that your energy state raises because you're doing what your body is truly designed to do - which is move. In moving, your blood flows faster, your energy vibrates higher and this increase in kinesthetic energy ignites The Law of Attraction. As you train this process, the body adapts to making this physiological increase in metabolism (the production of energy) your new normal and emitting high vibrations actually becomes a part of your DNA. The more you train, the more you program your body to produce radiant levels of positive energy.

Emotionally, developing a relationship with yourself is the inner work to fulfillment that so many people avoid. The journey is not easy and requires many challenging lessons that most people don't know how to overcome. The strongest leaders have fought these inner battles and use their experience to show up more powerfully to teach others. With the chaos of life, it can be hard to know where to start your inner work, but you can begin to learn many life lessons through the process of training. When exercising, you learn to what capacity you can push yourself, you learn about what you like, you learn about what you don't like. Through commitment and achievement, you learn about your state of mind and truly get connected to a deeper part of you. This emotional awareness is different than kinesthetic awareness. This connection ignites The Law of Attraction because you learn about yourself enough to decide what defines your true alignment - what is the true art to your fulfillment. Alignment is living life by your terms and realizing this truth is what feels best for all of us. Again, understanding what makes you feel good raises your vibrations. The more emotionally aware you become, the more attractive you become. People love authentic, aligned leaders. They are trustworthy, strong and consistent. Exercise can push your limits, so as you continue to grow and overcome, the power of your alignment continues to get better and better.

Mentally, exercise is a great opportunity to challenge and evolve your mentality through preset intentions. The Law of Attraction states what comes to you will either be positive or negative based on your thoughts and focus. If you are wanting to call in positive experiences, people or things; you must focus on finding that confident vibration of You at a higher level. So, how can you find a vibration of a level you've never reached before? Set intentions of how you want to think mentally as a leader. Visualize who you want to be in the future. Imagine what you would be doing and how you would think. Now, decide that when you train, you're going to intentionally focus on these elements during your workout so you can strengthen that new thought and draw positive energy to reinforce this part of you.

For example, as a leader, you might want to practice starting tasks and finishing strong. Set this intention and actively internalize that thought throughout each exercise: "I am choosing to do this action and I will finish to the best of my ability." It may seem like just a thought, but here is the trick: Every time you observe an intention, and follow through on that intention, you reinforce that vibration within your body. Anything you do often eventually becomes normal in all areas of your life. So, every time you complete an exercise set, you can celebrate your accomplishment and flood this mindset with positive energy. Don't miss the opportunity to acknowledge your success. It might seem like a small win, but if you continue practice winning, you will naturally become a winner.

How you do one thing is how you do everything. Setting the intention to complete tasks may start in the gym, but I guarantee it will eventually trickle into how you treat everything else in your life. This stair-step process to manifesting your internal strength and confidence radiates from the inside, so that you become more attractive on the outside. Ultimately, you're training your psyche on how to be a more solid leader. Choose any intention, they all apply, and watch how it permeates into other areas of your life.

As a leader who exercises and elevates their energy through movement, you will find your ideal clients attracted to working with you. People will want to get to know you and the confidence that comes from this high vibration. People will want to be in your space because they feel your energy. They will want to know what it is you do differently and will follow you because they feel closer to themselves by being in your proximity. Like attracts like and your example is truly magnetizing. This is how self-care as a leader radiates out and influences others around you. Use exercise to strengthen your magnet and you will receive bigger and better desires more easily than ever before.

Again, though there is a science to success, fulfillment is an art. It's really hard to find yourself feeling fulfilled when your body is failing you. Exercise is one the many ways to connect with your body, but there are other ways to maintain your energy. Now is the time to make the commitment to keeping your vibrations high. Here are some things you can do right now to get yourself on the right track.

Movement

Know that just engaging in the next 3 or 4 days in some form of movement will take you a long way. I don't mean something drastic—I'm not even talking about something that involves a gym or a workout routine—just going outside for 20 minutes a day and walking around the block will begin to stir up your energy. After doing this for a while, you can start looking into programs—whether that be things you do on your own, or working with a professional. The most important thing to remember in the beginning is to not focus so much on the how. What you will find is that every type of exercise is the RIGHT answer! As long as it makes you feel fulfilled and helps you keep your vibrations high, then that is the exercise type for you. Just go for it!

Rest

As supplementation to the conversation of exercise in this chapter, we have to understand how important rest is. Rest is the key to all that we do. As we work at keeping our vibrations high, daily stamina will only last for so long. Each of us needs time to step back—to recharge our batteries—to rest, in the form of sleep, meditation, and even taking some time off from work and exercise. This is every bit as important as our daily routines because all of this is maintenance on our bodies, minds and spirit. Rest connects us deeper to ourselves and brings out our best version through self-reflection, recovery and passive rebuilding. Afterwards, we come back refreshed to do our work all over again!

Nutrition

If you think of your body as a machine, then you can begin to see how important the fuel is that we give it. Nutrition feeds the body and feeds the power behind all the work that we do. You can't drive a car if you don't give it gas. Simply, it's just how that machine works. To take it another step, if you had a high-class car, like a Lamborghini, you wouldn't fuel it with low grade gasoline. It requires the highest quality of fuel because it is a high quality machine. The same is true for your body. Put this together and this is how your body—and the Lamborghini—can run at the optimal level. By giving yourself the right kind of nutrients, water, and supplements, your body can work properly, keep your energy up, and give you that inner confidence that seeps out of you in your day-to-day life - ultimately breeding attractiveness.

Remember that everything good comes in time. As you apply each of these things, it will allow you to be the attractive leader that you were always meant to be. Positive energy correlates with high vibrations, magnetism and radiance!

The more energetic you are in life, the more attractive you truly are. We should want to be a person of high energy because that is what attracts the things and people that we want in business and in life. With this new definition, we should learn to not look at the physical aspects of people, but rather their energy. Especially our own.

This is the true definition of confidence - and confidence is attractive.

~Samantha Nichole
Find me on Facebook:
Samantha Nicole
memoirese@gmail.com

STANDARD OF CARE
SAMAN BAKHTIAR

There are over 260,000 personal trainers in the United States, with a growth prediction of more than 338,000 in 2018. This is great news for the millions of people in America that need or want a personal trainer, but it is also worrisome. The average personal trainer undergoes a brief online course where they are certified at the end and are able to start working with clients. Sounds great, right? Wrong. There is a huge problem with the current standards for personal trainers.

When it comes to the fitness industry, the standards are lacking. Testing that can evaluate your knowledge and skills, a curriculum, and board exams should be standard. The curriculum should be hands-on training, and you need to know the anatomy, physiology and biomechanics of the human body in order to properly advise your clients. Just like with any other medical profession, a degree, a practical exam, and licensing should be required. Wondering why?

Imagine going to the dentist. You go through your exam or procedure and by the end of the appointment, you find that the dentist has messed up your teeth. Lucky for you, you can make an insurance claim that will pay you and pay another dentist to cover your damages. There is no such thing in personal training. If your personal trainer doesn't understand the human body, or maybe they don't have enough experience to give you the correct advice, you could be left with injuries that are painful, and some can be permanent. Guess what? They don't have malpractice insurance. They don't have any way for you to find legal recourse, which means you're stuck with your injuries and bad advice. See the importance?

By implementing standardized testing, exams, hands-on training, and licensing just as a physician, dentist, or even a lawyer would do, you can have peace of mind in knowing that this person is trained, knowledgeable, and able to help you meet your fitness goals in a healthy and safe way. The thing is, you hear all the time that people are given the wrong advice, they're told to eat this way or that way, take a supplement or don't and the problem is, these individuals don't have the proper knowledge to give you advice about nutrition or fitness. A personal trainer needs to know anatomy, physiology, biomechanics, and functions of the muscles, nerves, all of it. They need to be able to advise you on proper form and proper progression otherwise you can develop injuries and even metabolic disorders.

I have been a personal trainer since I was 18 years old. My passion in the industry also led to me getting my masters in pre-medicine and nutrition, my doctorate from the Los Angeles College of

Chiropractic, and it also led me to becoming ACE (American Council on Exercise) and NASM (National Academy of Sports Medicine) certified. My training has allowed me to successfully start and run a successful fitness company that helps thousands of people meet their goals every year. My experience, my background and skills are what assures me that the standards are not high enough for people in the fitness industry.

The standards will raise with time, but in the meantime, if you're looking for a personal trainer, there are a few things you should consider first. The most important thing you need to do is to ask for the trainer's credentials. Know what kind of education and certifications they have.

Are they keeping up with continued education? Do they know what they are doing? The next thing is to look around and see what kind of results they have with their current clients. Interview a few of their clients, ask around, and look around to see how they are with their clients. How many success stories do they have? Ask them to pull out pictures and testimonials. That will go a long way to telling you what this particular trainer is all about. There are good trainers everywhere. But there are also bad trainers everywhere, so you need to research and ask questions before you commit to a trainer long term.

Know what your ultimate goal is before you find a trainer. What do you expect from the trainer? Be realistic with yourself and your expectations, but be sure you can meet those goals too. Not only is it important that you know the trainer's skills and education, but also, you need to be sure that your trainer's personality matches yours. Maybe you're looking for a trainer because you need motivation. If your trainer doesn't motivate you to show up, that isn't going to make you successful in your goals. If a trainer has all of the credentials out there, but can't motivate you, that's not good. Consider a free trial or two with the trainer, or watch how they train a few other clients. How do they interact with the client? Are they attentive? Are they paying attention? Or, are they eating a sandwich while the client is training!? These are important things to consider when choosing your personal trainer.

With people walking less, things like public transportation, planes, computers, all of the things that are making people less motivated to be healthy, people in the fitness industry can rise to the top of the game if they have the skills to motivate their clients, go the extra mile, have the proper credentials and give the proper advice and follow up.

Those with an eye on the money to be made are the ones that cut corners, give bad advice and cause problems for their clients. The fitness industry is growing, and those with the passion, like myself, will make it far. With proper training, education, licensing and passion, anyone can jump into the fitness industry and be a successful personal trainer.

~Saman Bakhtiar
You can train with us, or inquire about becoming a new franchise owner at: www.thecamptc.com

MASTER YOUR BODY AWAKEN YOUR TRUE VITALITY & SUSTAINABLE WELLNESS
RACHEL RICHARDS

We all have fitness goals. Often, when the goal is to lose weight and build muscle, we jump into a program. The programs are usually recommended by a friend or maybe you saw it online. You start off so excited to get into the program and you really try to work the program, putting in all of your effort, but after a little time passes, you find yourself wondering where are the results?!

All of the promises are there, all of the hype too. The problem is that just because something worked for someone else, doesn't mean that it will necessarily give you the same results. There are fundamental things you can do to figure out the right path for yourself. As a fitness coach, that's what I want to do for you.

For years before I became a fitness coach, I was a business coach. I wrote a manual for NCR, helping people to embrace excellence in all that they do. I wrote it to push people and motivate them to excellence. After I turned 40, I retired from business coaching and I started really looking at training because it was where my heart was. I did some work as a spin instructor, I got certified in weight loss training as well as the metabolic syndrome. I really began to find for myself, a channel for helping people with their overall wellness. I still teach business sales excellence, and it parallels so well with what I do now in the wellness industry, because there really is a synergy between our mind, our body, and our spirit. More than anything, what I really love to do is help people discover the mysterious animal that is nutrition.

There are so many programs out there, but what we have to do is get away from the trends and listen to our own bodies. We have to develop a methodology to build our own nutrition powerhouse. The nutrition for our bodies that will serve us the best is actually the building blocks of the body that you want. Make sense? You have to discover how your body prioritizes health. People become bored with fads and chase another one. That's part of the problem. The fundamentals and your individual body needs have to be the focus. You have to master your body's needs. Many people, I'll admit, myself included, get caught up in the statistics and then ignore the fundamental building blocks because the trend says to—they give up things that are time-tested, but you need that breakfast of champions. You need those building blocks to succeed.

One of my heroes, Coach John Wooden from UCLA. He has coached great athletes like Kareem Abdul Jabar and so many others. He started every season by having the team unlace their shoes, take them off, take off their socks, and have them work on how to put their socks on properly and how to re-lace their shoes. Coach Wooden was quoted as saying, "We will lose a whole lot of games, but we're not going to lose them to blisters from socks or from poorly tied or untied shoes."

People are walking around these days clinically dehydrated, and even though we know that gut health is paramount to sustainable fitness, most people are not on that path, and we have to anchor ourselves in the fundamentals. There are so many options around! Let's be honest, we all know sugar is bad for us. We have to realize the addictive nature of sugar, the swelling that it causes and that it leads to injury. We have to learn to use food as a tool.

When I first started out, I found a lot of information on Google. I didn't realize that Google was a sales marketplace. It isn't somewhere that we should base our decision making. Sometimes we have to look past the article we are reading and follow the dollar. Who wrote the article? Who sponsored it? What is the reason for the article? Where is the money going to go?

Sometimes, the information that you're taking in, isn't necessarily meant to actually increase your wellness or nutrition, but rather, it's a really well done advertisement for a product. I started to realize that I had to dive deeper. I started looking at things like Google Scholar, White Papers, things that are written or documented by people that have certifications in the industry and really focused on the truth behind nutrition. Here is the big secret that I discovered. A "Food Mood Journal". So, what works for me? What kind of things happen with the food that I'm taking into my body? How does it affect me physically? How does it affect my mood?

I'm not the kind of trainer that will go on to Google and find a generic answer for a client. I have to go on a journey with you to help you find that truth for yourself. A lot of people I know have shut down on the whole concept of nutrition and they really don't know what to do with food anymore. Is milk good for you, or is it not? Are eggs good? Are they bad? There are so many different theories and opinions out there so people find themselves skipping the nutrition end of things all together and just go to the gym and workout. There are so many universal truths and most of those come out from a food mood journal.

It's so easy to become distracted by the documentaries that we see of the successes that other people have. I have found myself in weird places, and I found it using the journal. I was living as a vegetarian but by taking in all of the vegetables, my critical carbohydrate level was too high, and that I was storing water as a result, which was creating problems with my system. It made me gain fat! I learned a lot from the mistakes that I made early on, and I want to help you to be able to discover what works for you. I want you to see the secrets behind the time-tested fundamentals so that you can take action on the right things for you. We all know that 70% of fitness is in the kitchen and only 30% is in the gym. A lot of clean eating, a little bit of strength training and a little bit of cardio is really the ultimate combination for overall health. People get discouraged because while the 30% can be perfectly articulated for you in the gym by coaches or instructions, who really knows exactly what to do with the 70%? It's overwhelming!

Let's think about some basics just for a minute. Your body has a prioritization schedule of its own. A human being can only live ONE MINUTE without hope—that's a healthy mind. Without hope, we're in big trouble, really. We can only go THREE MINUTES without oxygen—so we have to learn how to breathe properly. We can go THREE DAYS without water, so we really have to focus on hydration! Many of my clients, when I tell them that "This week we are just going to focus on taking in enough water" they look at me like I am crazy! They think it should be harder than that, but if you can master hydration, often you'll begin to see results with just that change. We can go about THREE WEEKS without nutrition. So the question to ask yourself is, how long can you go without movement? How long will it take to have an effect on you? As we take things in that order, hope, oxygen, water, and then nutrition, and follow it up with movement and exercise, we can create a sustainable program that works for you!

We want to create a framework that will get you results in a way that works for your body's needs to feel nourished, fulfilled and healthy. When I work with my clients, I make sure they take the priorities that their body dictates to them—to get familiar with the priorities—and then I help you along the journey so that you can live a healthy life. My mission in life is to awaken you toward true vitality and sustainable wellness. Together, we can make that happen.

~ Rachel Richards
channelmywellness@gmail.com
Find me and PM me on Facebook:
RACHEL MARIE RICHARDS

RELAXED AWARENESS
MOLLY KUBES

Life is busy. All of us have daily challenges things that are part of our day to day life. Often, it becomes so easy to focus on all the things that we have to do today that we miss all of the things that are actually happening right here in the now.

I am a Reiki master (a Japanese method of energy healing), Conscious Business Strategist, & Prosperity Priestess, helping women especially find energy alignment within themselves.

I encourage them to use things like yoga and meditation to help them in their spiritual journey. I love mentoring these wonderful women, whether it be in person, on retreats in Hawaii, or any of the other forms. The best feeling in the world is to be able to help them find, within their lives, that state of relaxed awareness that allows them the ability to be the best version of themselves. As we focus on our relaxed awareness, we can find a place of bliss in all of the things that happen as we move through our life.

I know how difficult finding that balance that can be. Several years ago, I was lost. A shy girl who really didn't have a good or easy time coping in public. I was very energetically sensitive and because of that, it made it very hard for me to connect. To dull this within myself, I turned to things like alcohol and drugs. It soothed the pain. I felt all too often, of not really being connected to people and often feeling the energy around them too deeply. This dive into alcoholism and drugs, was my downward spiral. I really dove into that lifestyle completely.

I looked at my life one day and I realized this was not how I wanted to live. To be honest, I wasn't really living at all. I wanted it to change, but I didn't know how. All the friends that were my life at the time; their life was the same as mine, filled with drugs and alcohol. I didn't know any different because I had never seen anything any different.

I remember though, out of desperation, I took that moment and I prayed. Now, whether you believe in God, Gods source, the universe, or the divine; you know what I mean when I talk about a moment where you just simply stop and ask for guidance. "I need help," I said, "to make a change and to not live this way anymore." The outcome of that moment was not what I expected.

I ended up really sick with digestive problems and food intolerances. I didn't really understand it or appreciate it at that time, but looking back, now I understand that my body was rejecting the alcohol and drugs. My body was forcing me from the inside out to make a change, making it so that I literally couldn't live that lifestyle anymore.

As I was dealing with the digestive problems and the other physical things that were happening in my life, I was blessed to find Yoga and Reiki. I remember falling in love with it, going full force from the very first moment I saw it. I will never forget walking into that very first yoga class and knowing instantly that was what I wanted to do. I wanted to be a yoga instructor. There were so many signs during that point of my life that were showing me how much I could do and the things that I could do to help people. Even though, at the time, while I was going through it, I didn't see those signs. I now know that all of them that I went through where some of the greatest gifts and had helped me to be able to dive deeply into the things that I now teach. It allowed me to dive into the spiritual side of my life and become powerful internally so that I can live externally; a happy and blissful life, and to find empowerment, joy, and bliss.

This is something that I love to share. It brings me great delight when I can inspire other people and help them find a way to connect to their spirit. More than anything, I encourage you, to find a place where you can cultivate the ability in your own self to live in a state of relaxed awareness, to be in a place where the day doesn't just get by you but that you really truly live in. To be able to find all the subtle nuances and really find the joy and happiness that can be a part of your everyday life. You have to take the time to go inward and connect to yourself, to that spirit that is inside of you. We have to let go of all of the societal norms, the things that our friends and our parents have put on us and just simply focusing on you.

What does it take for you to grow? You see, things manifest spiritually before they happen physically. We can heal a broken relationship in our spirit before the break is so severe that it can't be fixed because now it's out in the physical realm. As we begin to develop the means to really deal with things on a spiritual level, before they manifest in the physical, that's what allows us to thrive. There are so many ways to connect to spirit.

We live in such a day-to-day society. That is what I might call, much of a male energy, if you will, in the yin and yang. The yang energy; that is all about external action. What we have to learn is how to go into the yin to focus on the internal. Something as simple as just our breathing. Take a long-hold yoga position and hold that pose, just allows us to let go. This allows us to balance all of the outward energy that is so on us all the time with the very necessary inward. If you ignore your internal for too long you will burn out. The go-go lifestyle that so many of us live, will end that manifesting in illness.

It did for me. I didn't take the time to focus on my inward space until my body forced me to move into a place where I found balance. We can do something as simple as holding a seated forward position. That allows us to find that balance between the external and the internal; between what we are inside and the actions that we take on the outside. What we find is, as we go deep into that internal it stimulates our parasympathetic nervous response and allows our alpha brainwaves to become active and actually spark the healing for your mind, body, and spirit.

My recommendation to you is to just start simply. It doesn't have to necessarily be a specific yoga pose. Even just sitting in a comfortable position. Close your eyes and focus on something as simple as just your own breathing. Allow yourself to actively tune into this present moment by disconnecting from all the actions that you have to take. Simply listening to your breath, and being in touch with who you are on the inside.

With so much going on, it's easy to not allow ourselves to be in touch with what's actually happening now. With something as simple as a meditation walk; we can walk and focus on nothing but our breathing. Or perhaps looking down at our feet and watching as they move or seeing the wind blowing through the leave and the air. Really be in touch with this moment, to accept the gift of being in the present. When we live, in this moment, we can experience bliss. It's the only place we truly can.

Often we find ourselves focusing on the past. We look back at all the things that were, but in the end all that is going to is lead to depression. We are concerned about what it's going to bring, or what's going to come in the future. That results in anxiety, but by that simple inward focus, as you're walking or sitting, it allows you to be truly present and to shift your life. As you learn how to be present in your own life, you will find that you are also able to be present with the people that are the most important in your life. People like your spouse and your kids.

Meditation is not a difficult thing. Meditation simply means relaxed awareness. It's that intentional, going inward, for even just five to ten minutes a day with the goal of learning how to really truly be relaxed and aware. Spending just that five minutes in relaxed awareness in meditation, gives us the ability to manifest that relaxed awareness all the time in our life. We can cultivate it until it's where we live. Until things, simple things like, traffic problems, don't affect us. So, instead of yelling at the person who cuts us off; we can simply take a moment and realize that that is something we can expel. Getting angry for that reason is not something that is going to serve us. As a result, we become less reactionary, and much more present and at peace.

Relaxed awareness gives us the ability to show up in all that we do as the best version of ourselves. We've taken the time to invest in ourselves and to know who we are. My hope and want for you is to take just five to ten minutes a day to step away from all of the external activities in the world. Just get in touch with you. To spend that time living centered in your own personal, relaxed awareness.

~Molly Kubes
Reiki Master, Conscious Business Strategist, & Prosperity Priestess

Find out more about Molly:
http://infinitelyblooming.clickfunnels.com/priestess moneyascension

KEEP IT SIMPLE
BOB THOMPSON

Everyone has a passion in life, right? Something in this world that makes you smile, makes you happy, and brings so much joy to your life. Everyone's passion is different but I've found a way to make my passion shape my life.

If you're like me when you first discovered this, you went all in. Diving in blind. And, it changed you in some way. For me, it started when I was about 14 or 15 years old. I was 115 pounds, just skinny as a rail, but I had this deep desire to look like one of the guys on those action movies I couldn't stop watching. I wanted that muscular physique; but ultimately I wanted to change myself.

Without saying anything to anyone around me, I just started working out. I didn't tell anyone because I was afraid and embarrassed of how they would react. Would they tell me it's a waste of time? Look at me differently? Judge me for some odd reason because I wanted to make a change?

As a result, I didn't really make progress in the first two years. But, that didn't stop me. It didn't matter because I was really passionate about it, felt great doing it, and wanted to know everything I possibly can about it. I knew I could make the dramatic changes I wanted, I just had to figure out how to make it happen.

I've always been the "act first, think later" kind of guy. I didn't know anything about working out, like most other people, but that wasn't going to stop me. I loved working out and as an extension, everything related. Like nutrition. I knew that was a big key in changing my physique. So, I became obsessed with learning everything I could in that area as well. Ever since, I've really had a hunger for the knowledge and self improvement that I gained from the first time I stepped into my parents basement to workout. That fateful day led to my obsession and desire to know everything exercise; working out, nutrition, and recovery.

Naturally I went into personal training. I was a strength coach for a while, but by the time I was 24 years old I was ready to move on and by 25 years old I owned my first gym. A personal training gym that specialized in training athletes. This was great. However, two years in i came to a realization. I realized that although I loved helping an athlete get stronger, run faster, or improve their vertical jump, what I really enjoyed was helping others make a transformation like the one I had made. When I started working out I really had zero confidence and low self-esteem, all around just being really unhappy with how I looked, and I saw that same feeling from other people. Which made me want to work more with those who had weight to lose or a body transformation to be had. Two years after opening my first gym, I switched focuses on instead of training athletes I shifted my focus to helping those in need of weight loss or body transformations - helping them the same way fitness helped me.

The biggest problem I see people experience when coming into the fitness world is overwhelm. There's so much information out there that before or shortly after getting started, they feel even more confused and frustrated. As a result, they end up stopping before they start or soon after because of the multitude of options and the lack of simple and clear information.

We're in a state of information overload right now. Tens to hundreds of different ways, all preached to be the best, to achieve the same result. Where does one even start and how can they be sure they're even choosing the best option? Now it seems like they're no real actual solution to their problem and with such overwhelm we can become to paralyzed to even start.

Years ago, when I was fresh out of college, I was looking for a suit to wear to a wedding. All I knew was I needed a black one and it needed to fit. Prior to this, all I wore were gym shorts and t shirts. I'm a personal trainer over here, I didn't need much else. What I needed for that wedding, I felt was pretty simple and should be easy to fulfill. However, when

I walked into the store this all changed. The sales person pointed at the wall that felt as if it was a mile long and in response to my request for a black suit that fit, they let me know "There's a whole lot of suits you can look at." I remember feeling such a sense of overwhelm. Not only did I have no idea where to begin, but it was too much to take in at once, so I just walked out, after pacing up and down the wall receiving zero help but increasing my overwhelm.

The next store I visited, still feeling overwhelmed, I explained what I needed and they came back with three options. The overwhelm was instantly faded. I wasn't given a sea of options to figure out on my own, I was given three options with no loose advice that would work for me. I had the suit I needed. I had the solution to my problem. That same service is what everyone needs. Give clarity and provide a simple solution to what they need you need from the start. There is no confusion, no overwhelm and no fear.

Unfortunately, often I've found when someone walks into the gym they're met with something similar to that first experience. A sea of machines and no proper direction. A trainer trying to justify their degree and attempting to over complicate an explanation or a workout. Every here and there they're given some nutrition advice, usually go to go to google, but no simple guidance. And information on a ton of different diet options for them to look up more.

As a result, the fitness industry can be the exact reason a person who struggles to start doesn't get results. I have found is that fitness trainers and coaches are missing the mark with their client.

We need to understand what is the reason why a client doesn't enjoy going to the gym? Why are they not losing weight or continuing to gain weight? Why are they not passionate about making a change to living healthy? Is there a lack of understanding?

Learning and researching all the tools is important from a coaches perspective and we must be focused on how we can help our clients and our communities improve their health. Educating and teaching how to eat better, how to improve their workouts, how to recover better, to everything in between. We're getting bombarded with differing information every week. Often times contradicting what the piece last week just said, that we have to be able to be a buffer for what the person needs as well as what is accurate. Otherwise, it can become so complicated that people will literally feel they have no idea what it means to be healthy or the entire idea becomes overcomplicated.

Getting Back to Simple

If we can get back to 'simple' and we can create an environment where a person loves working out or eating right, they like what they're doing, and getting results, chances are, they'll stick with it.

Make exercise enjoyable. Make nutrition easy and simple. Teach in an easy and understandable way. Realize people don't really care about the biomechanics behind an exercise. Only to know if it's going to help them. It's great for a trainer to know it. But a trainer doesn't have to sound like a text book even the most fascinated with exercise science doesn't enjoy reading. Especially someone who really only cares about losing 80 pounds and reducing their risk of earlier mortality.

Everything I provide to my clients I do in a simple and easy to digest manner paired with a community of like-minded people who are on a path of healthy living that they can connect with. Following a program that truly works and gives the client all of the information they need is really key to a person's success.

Getting to the heart of the client's issues in terms of nutrition and exercise is the best way to set them on a favorable path. But sometimes the best advice and most beneficial is simply, 'Just do it'. Just get started. It's better to move than stay still. In order to make a massive change, there has to be massive action.

Now that you're moving, make nutrition simple. The reality is that in order to live well, along with exercise you have to eat a diet of nutritious foods and not junk. Eliminate processed foods. Drink water every day and make sure you're getting enough fruits, vegetables and lean proteins. Eating regularly enough to avoid putting not eating enough calories or binge eating because of hunger. Both are bad. If you eat too little, that muscle becomes your energy. If you binge, you generally are going to make poor choices. Start your meals by filling up on veggies, then protein, and finally the carbs. Your body is great at telling you what you need. Use your hands to determine portions.

There are millions of programs out there that have confused people. Honestly, finding an activity that you're actually going to do, something that gets your heart rate up and you're satisfied doing it, that's what you should be doing. Whether that's running, HIIT classes, biking, strength training, bodybuilding, or a combination of all of them, the best exercise is the one you're actually going to do nearly every single day.

Simply put, each person has to find something that they enjoy doing and keep doing it. If you're not enjoying the exercise or the nutrition plan, the chances of you sticking with it are slim. Working out every day in a way that is sustainable is also important. With real guidance, you can overcome the fear that is very real to each person - changing habits is hard! We're all scared to make the changes, what if we don't succeed? What happens with this overwhelm and fear is that we tend to make excuses. Once you start making the excuses, the probability of sticking to the plan drops considerably.

Be Committed

Here's the thing. Being committed to the program is essential. Sounds self-explanatory, yeah?

 So how do you get committed to the plan? First, ask yourself: What do you want to happen? What is your goal? Why is it important that this happens? We have to move past the fears and begin to see success. Find out your why.

It is going to take big changes. It isn't going to happen overnight and it is going to take a complete and total program that allows you to change your habits every day. This will be hard. This will challenge you and make you want to quit. Knowing your why will keep you focused.

Keep it Simple! You do not need to workout two or three hours a day, start with 45 minutes a day or three 15 minute workouts every day, and start with a simple and easy to prepare nutrition plan that will make the requirements easy to meet. Being clear with what action to take is the only way to set yourself up for success, and prevent the overwhelm that can destroy your dedication to the plan.

For each person reading this now, the things that work are support, encouragement, and motivating to keep going, and remember to Keep it Simple.

~Robert Thompson
CEO legiontransform.com
Instagram - @bob_thompson1
For anyone wanting to start their own franchise:
legionfranchise.com

EMPOWERING FITNESS PROS
(A Message for Fitness Entrepreneurs)
ANTHONY STEEL

For those of you that know me, you know that I've spent some years working both as a trainer and then as a gym owner, but as my business continues to transform, what I have found is so exciting!

In moving from owning a gym to being a consultant for gym owners, I have been able to help over 160 owners begin to see really effective ways to bring prospects into their business. Now I get to help gym and boot camp owners all throughout the USA, from California to New York, and even out in France and the UK.

The problem that we have found in the fitness industry is that rather focusing on IMPACT, fitness pros can sometimes tend to focus too much on "growing membership" and forget that each member is an individual.

If we, as professionals stop focusing on the individual and their experience and results, we could be doing the entire fitness industry a huge disservice.

In order for a gym to effectively impact people we have to design systems that intentionally and authentically show our clients that we care about them and their results - *because we do!* For those fitness instructors that have turned business owners, I urge you to stay connected with WHY you became a fitness pro in the first place.

If it's like most coaches I speak to, you started in this field because your life was transformed in a deep and profound way by fitness. In my opinion, this is why you're the best possible solutions for others. But just because you're passionate about fitness doesn't mean you're going to have the greatest impact because you shouldn't be the best kept secret in your community.

If you are that passionate instructor I would love to see you move from working IN your business to a place where you work ON your business so you can dig deep inside of your community and become the go-to gym, delivering the best results and experience in your area.

One of the gym owners we consult in our Detox Client Generator family, Joey
Salipetro, in Davie, Florida was on the brink of losing it all. Before working with us Joey, the owner of Warrior Fitness, had an 800 Square foot gym, he was paying $4k a month in ad spend to acquire clients and on top of it
he was paying thousands a month to a business coach. Not to mention breaking up with his fiance of

5 years, tearing his bicep muscle while training, and being hit with the pneumonia!

I found Joey in the Summer which in our industry is almost always the months where fitness pros hang on for dear life and we hope to keep our lights on and keep up with overhead expenses until September when it starts to pick up again.

Joey couldn't wait that long as he just signed on a 5,000 square foot facility. Joey needed something to work fast. He jumped on our program, got to work, and within 21 days he signed up over 75 people. By the end of the challenge he converted 45 into ongoing clients which added over 5k monthly to his EFT.

Because that worked out so well Joey ran another challenge, this time a 28-day challenge. He executed our "No Ad Spend Rabbit Hole System" and acquired over 50 people with absolutely zero ad spend.

Within a month and half he brought his membership to over 150 members
and now I'm happy to say he just signed the papers on location number 2.

What did this mean for Joey?

This meant a passionate fitness pro who loves what he does can continue to impact his community instead of closing his doors due to a tanked business.

…And along the way, as Joey grew, by working with us and staying connected to the reasons he started in fitness in the first place he knew the importance of treating each member as an individual.

I absolutely love what I get to do. To see gym owners with a smile ear to ear while no longer being the best kept secret or having to spend their very last dime on high-priced business coaches or thousands of dollars on ads makes me happy.

If you or someone you know wants to be the best UN-kept secret in their town, have them contact us.

~Anthony Steel
www.wayoflifetransformations.com
anthony@wayoflifetransformations.com
Find Anthony Steel on Facebook
www.wayoflifeconsulting.com

www.ingramcontent.com/pod-product-compliance
Lightning Source LLC
Chambersburg PA
CBHW061726250726
48657CB00002B/800